I'd like to dedicate this guide to everyone who made it possible for me to attend my medical elective

Introduction

Planning my medical elective was a stressful albeit exciting process. Being a person who enjoys planning, naturally, I began organising it over a year before I was due to embark on, what turned out to be, an incredible experience and one I am unlikely to forget.

The idea of planning an entire clinical placement seemed daunting initially as, I felt there to be a lack of resources to help plan elective for the more recent medical school cohorts.

A quick internet search on electives revealed all the companies that offer their services to help you secure a placement, however, a look at their eye-watering fees left me with a bitter taste.

I was determined to work on an affordable guide that allowed me to share the process of planning an elective. I've used my personal journey, along with the obstacles I encountered and the subsequent troubleshooting that took place, that made it possible to attend my dream placements. This guide has been written in a simple and informal style, like seeking an opinion over a cup of coffee. I'm hoping this aids, and eases, the process of planning your elective.

The structure of this guide, including the topics that will be covered, is as follows:

- What is an elective?
- Where do I start?

- Securing contact details
- Reaching out
- Funding
- Before your elective
- Final words
- Email and Letter templates
- Checklist to help with the administrative element.

Lastly, I've also included a section to take notes, it's located at the back of the guide and may be useful to scribble any thoughts you have as you go along. Hope you like reading this as book much as I enjoyed writing it!

What is an Elective?

An elective is a medical placement that is often undertaken in the final year of training and lasts up to 8 weeks in a country of your choosing. Most medical schools allow you to use that time flexibly once you've fulfilled a certain number of weeks undertaking an elective.

The main objective of an elective is to hone further the capabilities, developed at medical school, in an environment other that the one you completed your training in. Students are encouraged to choose a placement in their field on interest, this can be a UK-based or an international elective. The vast array of options to pick from can make this process an overwhelming and tedious one.

A well-organised placement can go a long way in helping to develop your portfolio for your chosen specialty, thereby highlighting the importance of planning ahead.

Where do I begin?

The first question to ask yourself is where you could see yourself undertaking a 4-8 weeklong placement.

Would you like to travel and experience a different healthcare system or prefer to stay within the United Kingdom?

Would you prefer a large hospital or private clinic in cosmopolitan city or perhaps something in a developing nation?

Do you have a set budget? I speak more on this in the Funding section of this guide.

International electives provide you with the perfect well-timed escape after your final set of medical school exams. They also allow you to explore another healthcare setting, that is especially handy if you've been considering the idea of relocating as a way to 'test the waters' before you make the decision. However, it is important to acknowledge the language spoken at country you wish to pursue your elective in, as it would help further decide if there was a preference for an English-speaking location, thereby guiding your search further.

Having said that, an UK-based elective would also provide you with an incredible opportunity to network and grasp a better understanding of the training route after speaking with doctors about factors ranging from portfolio requirements to work-life balance.

From the very early days of medical school, I had always envisioned undertaking my elective placement in New York City. This helped make the decision process easier and I could then move onto the next step – the speciality.

Some students may find it more helpful to pick their field of interest before settling on a destination, this is an equally suiting way to go about the process. Go with what works well for you.

If you intend on choosing the country before the speciality, like I did, my advice would be to avoid setting eyes on a specific field early on, rather keep your options more generalised. This may sound counterintuitive at first and warrants an explanation – most fields in medicine can be grouped into being either medical or surgical, this is largely governed by the way training programmes are structured across the UK, there are some exceptions, such as ophthalmology and neurosurgery, they have their own run-through training pathways.

For most of medical school, I was set on pursuing cardiology as a career route however, as I progressed through the course, work-life balance, for the most part, seemed a strong deterrent factor and prompted a look at possible alternative speciality, especially given the demanding nature of their job. However, this thought was still in its early days, and I still insisted on trying to organise an elective in cardiology in New York City.

Securing Contact Information

A useful start would be to ask your medical school if they have any existing relations with hospitals, such as Visiting Student Learning Opportunities™ (VSLO®) program. Unfortunately, my medical school did not participate in such programs however, they had a reservoir of contact details from electives undertaken by cohorts previously. Contacting your medical school to obtain relevant information of such nature is an excellent starting point.

If you fall in the same position that I did, there are several websites, such as RocketReach, that give you access to the most efficient ways to get in touch with potential doctors who would be able to host you for the duration of your elective. This allows you to access the most up-to-date emails that will come handy to send your initial email.

Reaching Out

Despite having the contact details, it is still up upon you to make that initial contact. In this section, I will be sharing some of the tips I used to secure my placement.

The best way to start is by drafting an email. This is usually what first draws the attention of a potential elective host, keeping it brief and succinct is key.

I also began updating my CV, adding more achievements, projects, and leaderships roles I had undertaken over the past few years at medical school. Alongside this, I also began drafting a 'letter of intent' – this can be a useful document that highlights your aims and objectives of your elective. *I've shared a template of this letter of intent and the initial email towards the end of this guide, they will need to be tweaked to suit your needs as some sections were specific to me.*

In the email, it's often worthwhile attaching the following: (1) your CV, (2) the letter of intent and (3) a letter of recommendation from your university (on headed paper) as it gives the additional option for the physician to explore your interest in further detail. For instance, many doctors in the US were unfamiliar with the purpose of medical electives and clarifying this could perhaps put you in a better position to receive a response.

The letter of recommendation is helpful as it confirms your enrolled onto a medical school and are a registered student in good standing. This should be easy to request from your medical school.

Despite all your best efforts, you may not hear back right away. It's important to know when to chase these emails, given that doctors may be busy and could need a nudge to respond. Having said that, it's equally important to establish when a lead may not be interested.

As mentioned earlier, I was initially looking to pursue an elective in cardiology however, after months of emailing, I was unsuccessful as I failed to receive any responses. This prompted me to explore other specialties that shared a similar route, such as haematology – this field requires trainees to undertake a period of training in Internal Medicine, similar to a possible route to becoming a cardiologist in the UK. This is why, I felt that, being open-minded about the speciality of interest was useful when conducting your initial search.

Within a few days, I had secured an elective in the field of haematology and things finally started to get exciting as I felt closer to achieving the goal, I had set out to do. However, I was notified of the charge that I'd have to pay, via an agency. At this point, I wasn't feeling particularly hopeful, and given the lack of responses thus far,

I went on to accept the offer. This increased the projected cost of my trip however, I was awarded a grant that helped significantly and I speak more on this in the funding section of this guide.

Towards the end of my final year, I had started to develop a glowing interest in ophthalmology.

With a few weeks of my elective left to spare, that I initially intended to use as a break, I began the process of trying to secure a short elective in with an ophthalmologist in New York City. I employed the same strategy as above and soon managed find a corneal surgeon who seemed interested in hosting me for as long as I intended to stay.

There were no costs in securing the elective ophthalmology and, after having done my elective, I now know that most doctors don't typically charge. An observation made during my elective was that doctors often welcome medical students, and those undertaking pre-med courses without a fee, as they are able to assist with various aspects of caring for the patients on a daily basis. Moreover, this tends to be of mutual benefit as you'll able to learn new skills and grow your portfolio whilst helping out.

In hindsight, I should've waited for more responses before securing the first elective placement and one I would've not been able to pursue it if it wasn't for the grant. I hope sharing these lessons learnt helps you persevere with contacting potential hosts until you've secured your desired placement.

Funding

Funding electives can be expensive, depending on where you intend on undertaking them, this can make UK-based electives more appealing. Identifying your budget early on not only allows you to plan within your means but also anticipate any amount you'd need to save up in advance.

International electives can involve a multitude of costs:

- Occupational health-based tests (such a chest x-ray to check for tuberculosis, antigen levels for MMR vaccine, Tetanus booster etc.) that you are expected to fund yourself.
- Malpractice insurance
- Visas
- Flights
- Travel insurance
- Accommodation
- Communing within the city for work/ leisure
- Food budget

Pre-elective health checks can be expensive, especially if you don't have your recent medical data available. The best place to obtain this, for me, was to contact occupational health at my placement hospital to inquire about the various tests I had as part of my induction at the beginning of my clinical years. This gave me more up-to-date information that, not only prevented me from having to book expensive blood tests due to having them done previously, but it also allowed me to relay the most accurate information to my host.

Ensure your travel insurance covers you for the entire duration of your stay. Most providers often offer cover for a single trip lasting up to 31 days in duration at a time. If your elective is longer than this, you may need to pay for an extension.

Once all arrangements have been confirmed in writing, submit plans to your medical school as some schools will need to approve plans and may also need a risk assessment to be submitted. The risk assessment may ask questions such as: how you intend to deal with clinical risks (causing injury to you or to patients), what the HIV prevalence rate is in the country you are travelling to and what their PEP policy is at your placement along with what medication you'll have access to in the event of a possible exposure etc. Gathering this information as early as possible will give you sufficient time to obtain all the relevant details from your host.

In terms of reducing costs, it is also useful to check with your current medical indemnity provider, such as the Medical Defence Union (MDU), to see if they would be able to provide similar coverage for the duration of the elective. Fortunately, I could request a letter online with my provider at no added cost so this work well in reducing further expenditure.

Lastly, I had researched elective grants to see if I was eligible to apply for any, especially given how expensive New York City is known to be. The information on all available grants and bursaries is freely available online and it's worthwhile gathering this data to explore potential funding options. It should be noted that most grants and bursaries will need a confirmed arrangement in place when applying for funding.

Final year can be a stressful period and applying for grants can take a while due to the paperwork involved. I utilised elements from my letter of intent to request to be considered for funding, I was successfully awarded a speciality-specific grant that helped fund my elective significantly. It also worked well as it has been an incredible additional to my portfolio, it allows me to obtain 'points' for when I apply for my training application in my chosen speciality in the UK. I'd recommend applying for any available grants as they can be beneficial in both the long and short-term.

All the information mentioned above, and the process thus far, has been summarised in a flowchart on the next page. Please also refer to the checklist of documents that may be helpful to tackle the administrative element once an arrangement has been made with a suitable host (at the end of this guide).

Flowchart: Securing Your Elective

Where would you like to do you elective: nationally or internationally

↓

Would you prefer a large hospital or private clinic in cosmopolitan city or something in a developing nation?

↓

Decide on your budget

↓

Decide on the specially, refer to the relevant section of the guide to help with this.

↓

Contact your medical school to check for any programs they participate in/ any information from previous cohorts.

↓

If still unable to find something, try websites like RocketReach, to help find contact details of potential hosts.

↓

Draft an email to send out along with a letter of intent (see templates for inspiration)

↓

Email medical school to ask for a letter of recommendation to confirm you're a registered medical student in good-standing.

↓

Send the emails and await responses.

↓

Before confirming your arrangement, speak to your host about: aims and objectives, what an average day looks like, how hands on the placement will be, other requirements such as USMLE etc. (see my elective check list for more information).

Before Your Elective

Setting aims and objectives before the elective is a good way to direct what you're hoping to achieve.

Some hosts may like to schedule a video call, whereas some may prefer to communicate solely via email, these are both great ways to convey your goals before you're due to embark on your elective. Discussing these in advance allows the host to involve you in aspects that you're more interested in. For instance, due to an interest in ophthalmic surgery, the doctor shared her surgical schedule, this allowed me to observe an array of procedures, ranging from a routine cataract surgery to more recent cutting-edge procedures in the field.

I was also interested in networking and was invited to events such as a Women in Ophthalmology dinner during my placement too. Furthermore, I got to explore newer treatments in the market, in both haematology and ophthalmology, as I had the opportunity to speak to pharmaceutical industry representatives, who had been visiting the offices for the day, to discuss the future of medicine in the fields.

This section is specific for anyone looking to undertake a placement in the US. The USMLE is often an exam sat by students looking to obtain a licence to practise medicine in the US and, it isn't an exam I had ever taken. When speaking to the doctors, from both electives, I asked in advance if they were happy to host me despite not having sat this exam. Both doctors did not require the USMLE. My advice would be to avoid worrying about the USMLE and seeking clarification early on in the process.

I'd also recommended to discuss what an average day looks like and what your role would be before the start date.

Some doctors often have students play an active role and may expect you to undertake activities such as: assisting with working new patients up (I did this in both placements), scanning (I conducted ocular scans of patients before they were due to be seen by the ophthalmologist), setting up infusion lines etc. Such opportunities provided me with an encouraging environment to gain new skills and pushed me out of my comfort zone, thereby enabling further development from a professional standpoint. Having said that, it's important to always discuss your level of clinical competence, act within in throughout and to ask for help as needed.

Discussing paperwork in advance is also helpful as it gives your host plenty of time to fill out any necessary forms that are needed by your medical school to confirm attendance. Alongside this, introducing the idea of a letter of recommendation halfway through your elective would be a great opportunity as, if mutually agreed, it gives your host sufficient time to assess you and compose the document.

Final Words

Planning my elective went a long way in making the experience a pleasant and memorable one.

I thoroughly enjoyed both placements as I had the opportunity to network, understand the healthcare system in the US, learn new skills and techniques, and grow as a professional, these experiences will stay with me for years to come.

I hope my guide has equipped you with the necessary tools to help you secure yours.

Template: Initial Email

Dear Dr X

Hope you are well.

Introduction: My name is X, I am an X year medical student at X, United Kingdom and will complete the course and qualify as a doctor in X. As part of the undergraduate medical course, we have the opportunity to undertake an elective placement abroad in a speciality of our choosing.

Explain your goal: Through my time at medical school, I have developed an interest in the field of X and wondered if it would be possible to undertake a X week-long program with yourself, please. I believe, this experience will allow me to hone further my clinical capabilities...(and a short sentence on how this will be beneficial)....in the field of X.

Attachments: I have attached the following:

- a letter of recommendation from my university
- a letter of intent: stating my aims and objectives
- my CV to give an insight into my qualifications, projects, and prizes....
- additionally, I am happy to provide any other documents needed such as my medical indemnity that allows me to undertake this experience.

Sign off: I would like to thank you in advance and hope to hear from you soon.

Many thanks
X

Template: Letter of Intent

Full Name
Current address

Dear Dr X,

Introduction: My name is X, I am a 4th year medical student at the University of X, and will complete the course and qualify as a doctor in X. As part of the undergraduate medical course, I have the opportunity to undertake an elective placement abroad. Through medical school, I have developed an interest in the field of X and wondered if it would be possible pursue this at ....

By my elective start date, I will have completed clinical teaching and experience in the following specialties...

This paragraph focuses on how you gained an initial interest in the chosen field: Prior to commencing my course in Medicine, I did an undergraduate degree in X. It was here that I initially gained an interest in X, this prompted me to undertake a course on the X (briefly described how it helped). Undergoing clinical placements at medical school allowed me to develop this interest further in the form of experiences such as the opportunity to observe outpatient clinics as part of my X rotation.

Discussing your projects/ audits in chosen field etc: I am currently working on a project in X: describe the project and possibly any explain changes implemented, mention if you re-audited etc.

If you haven't done any project in the area of interest: I have also worked on several projects outside the field of X that have discussed in further detail in the CV attached with this email and perhaps explain a bit about how they have helped in a brief statement, perhaps any key transferable skills gained?

Optional - Speak about your academic strengths/ awards: I have always been a hard-working student and performed well throughout the medical course, I currently hold a position in the X decile (if available) based on my academic performance since the start of the program. During this time, I also received awards at the university... Alternatively, perhaps share exam data on a specific module that relates to you elective.

Aims of elective: The aim of this elective is to hone further my clinical capabilities....in the form of this experience that will help me develop further as a scientist, and as a responsible professional for when I graduate medical school in X.

My objectives are: (list 3-4 objective and keep they brief and list them)

1. X
2. X
3. X
4. X

Sign off: I would like to thank you in advance and hope to hear from you soon.

Yours faithfully,
X

Checklist

This section should help you with the administrative aspect of your elective once an arrangement has been made with a suitable host.

- ○ Occupational health clearance, check if this is needed and if you have all the relevant documentation in place.
- ○ Medical indemnity
- ○ Check visa requirements.
- ○ Flights (if applicable)
- ○ Travel insurance (if applicable)
- ○ Accommodation (if applicable)
- ○ Cost of food/ travel calculated per day.
- ○ Search for all available grants and apply as early as possible.
- ○ Submit plans to medical school as some schools will need to approve plans and may also need a risk assessment

Notes

About the Author

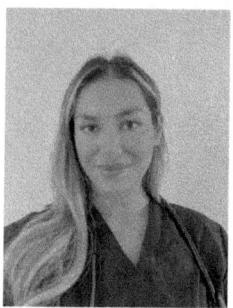

Arshi recently obtained a degree in Medicine, from the University of Buckingham, in June 2023. Prior to this, she graduated with a degree in Biomedical Sciences at St George's University of London in June 2018. She currently works as a doctor, completing her foundation training, within the Oxford deanery in the UK.

The medical elective was an experience Arshi had always looked forward to since her initial days at medical school. Electives are a great way to develop your portfolio in your desired speciality. With this guide, she hopes to share everything learnt, from the process of planning her elective placement, to make your journey a smoother sail.

This affordable guide comes equipped with a flowchart, a check list, and templates to help you secure your elective.